I0449235

LIFEWAVE PATCH TRAINING HANDBOOK

ISBN 978-1-300-89251-9
Fred Williford
Copyright@2024

TABLE OF CONTENT

CHAPTER1 3
   INTRODUCTION 3
CHAPTER 2 11
   The Principles Underlying
   LifeWave Patches 11
CHAPTER 3 21
   Varieties of LifeWave Patches
   and Their Purposes 21
CHAPTER 4 31
   How to Apply LifeWave Patches31
CHAPTER 6 49
   Guidelines and Optimal
   Approaches for LifeWave Patch
   Application 49
THE END 58

CHAPTER1

INTRODUCTION

LifeWave is a company dedicated to improving well-being through cutting-edge products that promote the body's innate healing abilities. Established in 2004, LifeWave is recognized for its innovative approach to wellness technology, especially with its non-invasive patches that utilize the body's energy systems. LifeWave's mission is to enhance overall well-being by emphasizing solutions that elevate both physical and mental health, providing products designed to boost energy, improve sleep quality, alleviate pain, and increase vitality.

At the heart of LifeWave's philosophy is the conviction that the body possesses the innate ability to heal and sustain itself when provided with the appropriate resources and surroundings. The company's method focuses on phototherapy, a natural and scientifically supported process that empowers the body to utilize its inherent energy. Through groundbreaking research and advanced technology, LifeWave strives to enhance well-being for all, inspiring individuals to embrace healthier lifestyles by harnessing their own biological functions. Today, LifeWave products are embraced by a worldwide community, encompassing athletes, health professionals, and individuals in search of natural, non-invasive solutions for daily health issues.

What Are LifeWave Patches?

LifeWave patches are adhesive applications intended for placement on targeted areas of the body, stimulating the body's inherent energy and wellness mechanisms without relying on pharmaceuticals or synthetic substances. Every patch is crafted with organic crystals that engage with body heat and light to activate particular cellular functions. Through a technique known as phototherapy, LifeWave patches stimulate specific biological responses, including enhanced energy production and better cellular repair, by gently and non-invasively applying light.

LifeWave patches function in a manner akin to acupuncture, focusing on specific areas of the body to enhance overall well-being. However, rather than using needles, LifeWave patches function by reflecting particular wavelengths of light back into the body. The patches feature a combination of natural components encapsulated in an organic crystal framework. When placed on the skin, the body's infrared heat triggers the patch, which subsequently reflects specific wavelengths of light that encourage various biochemical processes. Every type of patch is crafted to elicit a unique physiological response, targeting particular health requirements.

The technology operates through a non-invasive method, ensuring that nothing penetrates the skin or enters the bloodstream. Instead, it harnesses the body's energy to stimulate various processes that promote health and well-being. This approach makes LifeWave patches an attractive option for individuals seeking non-invasive, drug-free solutions to improve their well-being.

 Advantages of Utilizing LifeWave Patches

LifeWave patches offer numerous advantages that span various aspects of health and well-being. Here are several important benefits that LifeWave patches provide:

 1. Pain Relief and Inflammation Reduction - IceWave Patch: A widely recognized patch from LifeWave, the IceWave Patch is specifically crafted to address and ease discomfort. IceWave operates by activating specific areas on the skin, assisting the body in minimizing

inflammation and easing discomfort through natural energy pathways instead of relying on chemical solutions.
- Advantage for Individuals with Persistent Discomfort: Chronic pain can be incredibly challenging, and IceWave offers a reliable option that avoids the risks associated with opioids and other pain-relief medications that may lead to dependency. Individuals experience alleviation from discomfort in muscles, joints, and headaches, enabling them to engage in their daily routines with ease.

2. Boosted Vitality and Endurance - Vitality Patch: LifeWave provides the Vitality Patch, designed to elevate energy levels by enhancing fat metabolism and maximizing oxygen use within the body. This patch is a popular choice among athletes and those who lead active lifestyles, as it enhances endurance and boosts performance.
- Advantage for Daily Tasks: By boosting natural energy levels, the Energy Enhancer Patch aids in maintaining physical activity and can enhance mental clarity and concentration. This is particularly advantageous for those facing significant physical or mental challenges, along with individuals experiencing low energy levels.

3. Stress Reduction and Mood Enhancement - Aeon Patch: LifeWave's

Aeon Patch is designed to alleviate stress and encourage a sense of calm. It functions by harmonizing the autonomic nervous system, which governs the body's reaction to stress. By soothing this reaction, Aeon aids in alleviating signs of anxiety and tension.

- Advantage for Psychological Well-being: Stress is a prevalent concern that affects bodily health, emotional state, and general wellness. Aeon provides a holistic method for managing stress, promoting calmness and focus without inducing any sedative effects, ensuring users remain alert and energized.

4. Enhanced Sleep Quality - Silent Nights Patch: LifeWave's Silent Nights Patch aims to promote natural sleep rhythms, improving both the quality and length of your rest. The patch promotes the body's inherent ability to produce melatonin, aiding individuals in achieving quicker sleep onset and waking up rejuvenated.

- Advantage for Sleep Issues and Disorders: Rest is essential for peak well-being, and interruptions can result in various health problems, ranging from compromised immunity to psychological difficulties. Silent Nights offers a gentle, holistic approach to enhancing sleep quality, eliminating concerns about dependency or adverse effects linked to typical sleep aids.

5. Dermal Wellness and Recovery - Y-Age Carnosine Patch: The Carnosine Patch promotes the swift repair and renewal of skin cells, providing advantages not just for the skin but also for tissues and muscles. It has demonstrated encouraging outcomes in enhancing recovery from injuries and promoting skin elasticity.
- Advantages for Older Adults and Rehabilitation: As individuals grow older, the process of cellular renewal diminishes, resulting in the appearance of wrinkles, a decrease in the speed of wound healing, and a loss of skin elasticity. Carnosine may aid in enhancing recovery times and preserving skin vitality, making it a great choice for individuals aiming to support youthful skin and quicker recovery.

6. Detoxification and Immune Support - Glutathione Patch: LifeWave's Glutathione Patch supports the body's detoxification processes and enhances immune function. Glutathione is a powerful antioxidant that neutralizes free radicals and protects cells from damage, essential for maintaining overall health.
- Benefit for Immune Health: In the current landscape, where contact with harmful substances is prevalent, enhancing the body's natural cleansing systems is crucial for well-being. The Glutathione Patch aids in eliminating

toxins from the body and enhancing immune function, offering support for both immediate and sustained well-being.

7. Enhanced Appetite Regulation and Weight Control - SP6 Complete Patch: SP6 Complete aids in regulating appetite and promotes effective weight control. By activating targeted areas on the body, SP6 Complete aids in harmonizing hormones linked to hunger and fullness. - Advantage for Managing Weight: For those facing challenges with cravings or weight concerns, SP6 Complete provides a helpful alternative that avoids the use of dietary stimulants or appetite suppressants, presenting an effective and sustainable method for managing weight.

LifeWave patches provide a groundbreaking, non-pharmaceutical method for enhancing health and well-being through the utilization of light therapy. Offering a range of patches tailored to address specific requirements, LifeWave presents choices for those seeking to alleviate discomfort, enhance vitality, diminish stress, promote restful sleep, support skin wellness, detoxify, and regulate weight—all by harnessing the body's innate energy mechanisms. LifeWave's emphasis on gentle, safe, and effective solutions positions it as an excellent option for those seeking a comprehensive approach to improved well-being. This introduction lays the groundwork for grasping the distinct advantages of LifeWave patches, equipping new users to seamlessly integrate these patches into their wellness practices with assurance and insight.

CHAPTER 2

The Principles Underlying LifeWave Patches

LifeWave patches utilize advanced technology that taps into the body's innate ability to heal through light therapy, a method extensively researched and applied in healthcare to support recovery and improve physical capabilities. In this section, we'll delve into the scientific principles behind LifeWave patches, examining the fundamentals of light therapy and the clinical research that validates their efficacy. We will also address frequently asked questions regarding the functionality of these patches and what contributes to their safety and reliability as a wellness option.

Exploring Phototherapy: The Mechanism of LifeWave Patches and Their Interaction with the Body's Innate Energy

Light therapy, also known as phototherapy, utilizes particular wavelengths of light to trigger biochemical processes within the body. This principle is frequently applied in therapies for skin conditions, seasonal mood fluctuations, and alleviating discomfort. Light therapy is effective as our bodies can take in and use specific wavelengths to activate cellular functions, similar to how exposure to sunlight encourages vitamin D synthesis in the skin.

LifeWave patches utilize a distinctive approach to phototherapy, functioning by reflecting particular wavelengths of the body's own infrared energy back into the skin, rather than emitting light themselves. Every patch contains organic nanocrystals that are uniquely designed to reflect light within the infrared and near-infrared spectrum. When a patch is applied to the skin, it interacts with specific wavelengths of light that are taken in by cells, initiating a range of natural biochemical reactions. The emitted wavelengths are influenced by the unique design of each patch, as various patches aim to address distinct health and wellness objectives.

1. Non-Transdermal Mechanism: LifeWave patches operate on a non-transdermal basis, indicating that they do not deliver any chemicals or substances into the body. This approach offers a safer, more holistic means of activating the body, free from the side effects often linked to conventional

medications or supplements.

2. Activation of Pressure Points: The patches are frequently applied to specific pressure points, akin to the practice of acupuncture, yet they do so without the use of needles. These areas on the body are linked to particular internal systems or functions. By stimulating these areas, LifeWave patches promote the body's natural ability to unleash its own restorative energies.

3. Light Interaction and Biological Response: LifeWave technology is founded on the principles of light interaction with living tissues. When light energy interacts with cells, it can elevate mitochondrial function, amplify ATP synthesis, and improve the processes of cellular repair and regeneration. The patches function by amplifying these light-sensitive mechanisms, inherently bolstering the body's capacity for self-repair, pain management, and overall health maintenance.

Research and Findings: Empirical Backing for LifeWave Patch Efficacy

LifeWave's dedication to scientific validation has resulted in numerous clinical studies, demonstrating favorable outcomes in aspects like pain alleviation, enhanced energy levels, and better sleep quality. Here is a summary of several important research findings that demonstrate the efficacy of LifeWave patches:

1. Pain Relief and Anti-Inflammatory Effects - Research on LifeWave's IceWave patch has shown notable decreases in discomfort and swelling. In a controlled study, participants showed a significant reduction in pain levels while using the IceWave patch, with no side effects reported. The IceWave patch promotes the body's inherent energy movement, providing pain relief akin to traditional acupuncture while avoiding the discomfort of needles.

2. Enhanced Vitality and Endurance LifeWave's Energy Enhancer patch has been studied and shown to notably boost stamina and endurance. A study involving athletes revealed that individuals utilizing the Energy Enhancer patch experienced significant enhancements in their physical performance. The patch functions by facilitating the process of fat oxidation, thereby increasing the availability of energy. The enhanced vitality arises from the body's inherent metabolic functions instead of relying on stimulants, ensuring this is a secure choice for prolonged energy levels.

3. Improved Sleep Quality - LifeWave's

Silent Nights patch, designed to enhance sleep, has demonstrated an increase in melatonin levels among users, leading to superior sleep quality. Research studies have shown that participants reported a notable enhancement in both the length and quality of their sleep, all while avoiding feelings of grogginess or reliance, in contrast to conventional sleep medications. This patch functions by enhancing the body's natural rhythm, the essential cycle of sleep and wakefulness, which is vital for attaining rejuvenating rest.

4. Support for the Immune System and Cleansing The Glutathione patch has demonstrated the ability to elevate glutathione levels, a powerful antioxidant in the body, by up to 300% within a mere 24 hours. Glutathione is essential for immune health and detoxification, helping neutralize free radicals and remove toxins from the body. Studies have indicated that regular use of the Glutathione patch can enhance immune function and provide greater protection against environmental toxins.
5. Cellular Repair and Skin Health - The Y-Age Carnosine patch, which targets cellular repair and regeneration, has demonstrated benefits for wound healing, muscle recovery, and skin health. Carnosine is a naturally occurring dipeptide that helps protect cells from

oxidative damage. In clinical trials, participants noted enhanced skin elasticity, diminished wrinkles, and quicker recovery from minor injuries, highlighting the patch's ability to bolster the body's inherent healing processes.

6. Improvements in Mental Function and Emotional Well-being The Aeon patch, crafted to alleviate stress, has demonstrated effective outcomes in diminishing anxiety and enhancing mood. This patch aids in harmonizing the autonomic nervous system, potentially diminishing the body's reaction to stress. Individuals involved in research have indicated experiencing increased calmness and enhanced focus, which may offer advantages for psychological well-being, cognitive abilities, and emotional strength.

These studies highlight LifeWave's dedication to wellness grounded in scientific evidence. Offering a non-invasive and natural approach to health, LifeWave patches present a scientifically backed alternative to conventional treatments, especially in pain relief, energy boosting, and immune system support.

Frequently Asked Questions about Patch Technology

While LifeWave patches are quite groundbreaking, it's completely understandable to have inquiries regarding their functionality, safety, and efficacy. Here are some frequently asked questions and their answers to enhance understanding of the principles and advantages of LifeWave patches.

1. What is the mechanism behind LifeWave patches if they do not penetrate the skin? - LifeWave patches are designed to be non-transdermal, which indicates that they do not transmit chemicals or medications through the skin. Rather, they function by bouncing particular wavelengths of light back into the body. This engagement with the skin's receptors activates particular biochemical processes that affect well-being, vitality, discomfort levels, and beyond.

2. How do LifeWave patches utilize light therapy? - Light therapy utilizes illumination to influence biological processes. The patches interact with the body's infrared heat, prompting it to generate particular biochemical responses. The responses are tailored based on the specific patch, as each patch's crystal structure is crafted to emit distinct wavelengths for focused advantages.

3. Is the use of LifeWave patches considered safe? - Indeed, LifeWave patches are considered safe for use. These methods are gentle and avoid the introduction of any substances into the circulatory system. Research has demonstrated that LifeWave patches are free from negative side effects and are suitable for individuals across all age groups. Nonetheless, like any health-related product, it's important to adhere to guidelines and seek advice from a healthcare professional if there are particular medical issues.

4. What is the expected timeframe for users to see results from LifeWave patches? - The duration required to observe outcomes can differ based on the person and the specific patch utilized. Certain patches, such as IceWave for alleviating discomfort, might offer instant relief, whereas others aimed at enhancing sleep or promoting detoxification could take several days to achieve their maximum impact. Numerous individuals observe enhancements in just the initial week of regular application.

5. Are LifeWave patches compatible with other therapies or medications? - LifeWave patches typically work well alongside other therapies, as they do not interfere with medications or treatments

that affect the circulatory system. It is important for individuals to seek guidance from their healthcare professional prior to using the patches in conjunction with other therapies, particularly if they have any pre-existing health issues.

6. Are LifeWave patches effective for all individuals? - As with any approach to well-being, personal reactions can differ significantly. Although numerous individuals encounter beneficial outcomes, elements like personal health condition, lifestyle choices, and particular health requirements can affect the results. LifeWave offers a variety of patches, enabling individuals to discover options that align with their specific health aspirations.

The principles underlying LifeWave patches integrate the body's inherent energy with the concepts of light therapy, providing numerous health advantages without resorting to invasive procedures or chemical substances. By reflecting certain wavelengths of light, LifeWave patches activate natural biochemical processes that may assist in alleviating pain, boosting energy levels, enhancing sleep quality, promoting detoxification, and more. Backed by clinical research and providing a safe, non-invasive approach, LifeWave patches present a distinctive option for individuals looking for natural, evidence-based wellness solutions. By grasping this cutting-edge technology, newcomers can assuredly investigate how LifeWave patches might cater to their unique wellness requirements.

CHAPTER 3

Varieties of LifeWave Patches and Their Purposes

LifeWave patches provide numerous advantages, including alleviating discomfort, boosting energy levels, enhancing sleep quality, and supporting detox processes. Every kind of patch is crafted with particular health objectives in focus, employing light therapy to activate the body's inherent biochemical reactions without relying on pharmaceuticals or synthetic substances. In this discussion, we will delve into the various categories of LifeWave patches, highlighting their distinct functions and the underlying principles that support each one.

1. Alleviation of Discomfort: IceWave Patch for Discomfort and Swelling

The IceWave patch is designed to alleviate both sudden and long-lasting pain, making it perfect for individuals seeking a natural, non-pharmaceutical solution for handling discomfort. IceWave patches function by harmonizing the body's energy pathways, potentially alleviating discomfort and swelling.

- How It Works: The IceWave patch employs light therapy to stimulate targeted areas on the body linked to alleviating discomfort. These patches are applied to specific points and engage with the body's infrared energy, activating the nervous system to reduce pain signals.
- Benefits: IceWave patches are especially useful for alleviating discomfort in the back, joints, muscle strains, and headaches. Research indicates that individuals often feel a swift alleviation of discomfort, frequently within moments of using the patches, and without the adverse effects typically linked to pain relief medications.

2. Vitality & Endurance: Patch for Elevating Energy Levels

The Energy Enhancer patch aims to boost physical energy, elevate stamina, and enhance overall vitality. It's particularly advantageous for competitors and individuals aiming to sustain steady vitality all day long.

- How It Works: This patch facilitates the process of utilizing fat within the body, enabling it to rely on fat as its main source of energy. This method, consequently, delivers a more consistent energy output throughout the duration. Similar to the other LifeWave patches,

the Energy Enhancer utilizes phototherapy to boost metabolic efficiency without depending on stimulants.
- Benefits: Research indicates that athletes utilizing the Energy Enhancer patch report increased stamina and better recovery after workouts. It is perfect for those seeking to enhance their vitality without the fluctuations and downturns linked to caffeine or other stimulants.

3. Stress Relief: Aeon Patch for Alleviating Tension and Encouraging Calmness

The Aeon patch aims to promote equilibrium within the autonomic nervous system, the component responsible for regulating stress reactions. By harmonizing this system, the Aeon patch aids in alleviating stress and encourages a state of tranquility.

- Mechanism of Action: The Aeon patch employs light therapy to facilitate a soothing response within the body. When applied to specific points linked to alleviating tension, it aids in lowering cortisol levels (the primary hormone related to stress) and promotes a feeling of tranquility.
- Benefits: Aeon is well-regarded for its effectiveness in handling everyday stress,

anxiety, and fluctuations in mood. Numerous individuals have shared that they feel an increased sense of focus and relaxation, with some noting a decrease in physical manifestations associated with long-term stress, including muscle tightness and exhaustion.

4. Rest Enhancement: Silent Nights Patch for Better Sleep Quality

The Silent Nights patch is expertly designed to improve sleep quality, assisting users in falling asleep more quickly and attaining a deeper, more restorative night's rest. This patch is particularly beneficial for individuals experiencing difficulties with sleep stemming from stress, anxiety, or inconsistent sleep routines.

- How It Works: The Silent Nights patch promotes the natural production of a hormone that plays a crucial role in managing the sleep-wake cycle. When placed on targeted areas of the body, the patch enhances the natural rhythms, assisting users in achieving restful sleep effortlessly.
- Benefits: Users report achieving a more profound and restorative sleep, free from the grogginess often linked to sleep medications. Silent Nights enables users to rise feeling rejuvenated and more aware. Research has demonstrated

enhanced sleep duration and quality with consistent application.

5. Skin and Wound Healing: Y-Age Carnosine Patch for Enhancing Skin Recovery

The Y-Age Carnosine patch is crafted to enhance skin vitality, support tissue regeneration, and safeguard cellular integrity. Carnosine acts as a natural protector for cells against oxidative harm, which can lead to aging signs and cellular deterioration.

- Mechanism: This patch emits specific wavelengths that promote the production of carnosine within the body, aiding in the regeneration and repair of tissues. Carnosine contributes to cellular well-being by safeguarding against free radicals and oxidative stress, factors that can hasten aging and harm the skin.
- Benefits: The Y-Age Carnosine patch is frequently utilized to enhance skin flexibility, diminish the appearance of fine lines, and accelerate the healing process of wounds. Individuals often discover it advantageous for recuperation following exercise, as it supports muscle healing and alleviates discomfort.

6. Detoxification: Glutathione Patch for Purifying and Enhancing Immune Function

Glutathione, often referred to as the body's primary antioxidant, plays a crucial role in detoxification and supporting immune health. The Glutathione patch aims to enhance glutathione levels within the body, providing support against environmental toxins, pollutants, and oxidative stress.

- How It Works: When placed on the skin, this patch enhances the body's ability to produce glutathione, essential for the detoxification of cells. Glutathione attaches to harmful substances in the liver and aids in their elimination, improving the body's inherent cleansing processes.
- Benefits: Consistent application of the Glutathione patch may enhance immune function, boost antioxidant defenses, and assist the body in eliminating toxins. Research has demonstrated a notable rise in glutathione levels among participants, potentially enhancing overall health and fortifying the body's defenses against diseases.

7. Additional Patches and Their Distinct Advantages

Alongside the previously mentioned patches, LifeWave provides a variety of additional patches, each designed with distinct advantages to address specific health and wellness requirements.

Nirvana Patch: Elevating Your Mood

The Nirvana patch is designed to uplift mood and support emotional wellness. This approach is particularly advantageous for individuals dealing with feelings of sadness, anxiety, or fluctuations in their emotional state. The Nirvana system features a patch and a supplement that work together to enhance the production of endorphins, often referred to as the body's "feel-good" hormone.

- Mechanism: The Nirvana patch activates the release of endorphins, fostering sensations of joy and tranquility. It functions by bouncing back certain wavelengths that engage with the body's biochemical processes to enhance mood in a natural way.
- Benefits: Users report a significant enhancement in emotional balance, a decrease in feelings of anxiety, and an overall sense of wellness. The integration of the patch and supplement provides a comprehensive method for enhancing mood while avoiding the adverse effects linked to traditional medications.
SP6 Complete Patch: Appetite Regulation

The SP6 Complete patch is crafted to assist in controlling cravings and balancing appetite, making it a superb choice for individuals focused on weight management and fostering healthy eating patterns.

- Mechanism of Action: The SP6 patch functions by focusing on specific pressure points linked to appetite regulation and hormonal balance. The patch's technology aids in harmonizing essential hormones linked to metabolism, potentially leading to diminished food cravings and improved management of eating behaviors.
- Advantages: Individuals frequently share that they feel a greater sense of mastery over their hunger, encounter reduced urges, and promote more nutritious eating habits. This patch is particularly beneficial for individuals who face challenges with emotional eating or find it hard to manage portion sizes.

X39 Patch: Activation of Stem Cells

The X39 patch represents one of LifeWave's cutting-edge innovations, aimed at enhancing stem cell activation and promoting comprehensive cellular well-being. Stem cells are essential for the body's inherent healing processes, and the X39 patch is designed to enhance the rejuvenation of these cells.

- How It Works: The X39 patch is designed to reflect wavelengths that stimulate particular peptides within the body, promoting the activation of the body's own stem cells into a more dynamic and restorative condition.
- Advantages: Participants have noted enhancements in skin vitality, heightened energy, quicker recovery periods, and a noticeable decrease in the visibility of scars and fine lines. This patch is especially favored by individuals seeking to boost their body's inherent capacity to heal and rejuvenate tissues.

Y-Age Aeon Patch: Rejuvenation and Relaxation

The Aeon patch focuses on alleviating stress, but it also offers advantages for maintaining a youthful appearance. By reducing inflammation and encouraging relaxation, Aeon fosters a harmonious stress response, which is advantageous for both mental and physical well-being.

- How It Works: Aeon employs light-based therapy to impact the nervous system, alleviate inflammation, and harmonize the body's reaction to stress. Chronic stress can speed up the aging process, making the Aeon patch's capacity to alleviate stress significantly beneficial for anti-aging initiatives.

- Benefits: Users of the Aeon patch frequently experience reduced signs of aging, a greater sense of tranquility, and heightened mental clarity. Consistent application can enhance a more vibrant look by reducing the impact of oxidative damage.

LifeWave patches are crafted to address various wellness requirements, including alleviating discomfort, boosting energy, promoting detoxification, and improving skin health. Every patch employs LifeWave's innovative phototherapy technology to naturally activate the body's healing mechanisms without relying on medications or supplements. With an expanding collection of research and many success narratives, LifeWave patches provide a practical, non-invasive method for enhancing overall wellness. By grasping the distinct roles of each patch, individuals can select the most suitable options to enhance their personal health objectives and enjoy the advantages of LifeWave's groundbreaking wellness solutions.

CHAPTER 4

How to Apply LifeWave Patches

Applying LifeWave patches correctly is essential for getting the most out of their unique health benefits. Each type of patch is designed with specific placement points and usage guidelines, tailored to the individual needs of users. In this guide, we'll cover general guidelines for application, specific instructions for each type of patch, and tips for maximizing their effects.

1. Basic Guidelines for Patch Application

Choosing the Correct Placement Location for Optimal Benefits

Choosing the correct placement location for each LifeWave patch is crucial, as the patches work through phototherapy on specific acupressure or meridian points on the body. Each patch has optimal placement spots that help activate its intended benefits.

- Recommended Points: LifeWave provides a placement chart for each patch that outlines the best positions on the body for application. These points are generally based on acupressure or meridian locations, which help target specific health concerns, whether it's pain relief, energy enhancement, or stress reduction.

- Personal Preference: While the recommended points yield the best results, users can experiment with different placements based on their individual responses. Some users find certain positions more effective for specific symptoms, so it's encouraged to track personal experiences with each placement.

- Common Points: Some patches, like the IceWave patch, are often placed on both sides of a painful area for symmetry. Patches like the Aeon can be applied to specific points on the wrist or behind the ear for stress relief, as these areas are close to nerves or acupressure points that respond well to the patch's signals.

Duration for Patch Application and Suggested Frequency of Use

For optimal outcomes, adhering to the suggested duration and frequency of use is essential. Various patches might present slightly different instructions, yet common practices encompass:

- Daily Use: The majority of these patches are crafted for everyday application, particularly those focused on providing ongoing advantages such as increased energy, alleviation of stress, or detoxifying effects.

- Wear Duration: Generally, LifeWave patches are applied for a period of 12 hours. Following a duration of 12 hours, it is advisable to take them off to provide the body with a recovery phase prior to reapplication.

- Frequency: Many patches are generally safe for everyday application, but it can also be advantageous to incorporate brief pauses from their use. For instance, individuals may utilize patches for five to six days each week, followed by one to two days of rest. This interval provides an opportunity for the body to rejuvenate and may assist in avoiding reduced sensitivity to the impacts of the patches.

Instructions on Cleaning Skin Before Application

Preparing the skin before applying LifeWave patches is essential for proper adhesion and effectiveness:

- Clean and Dry the Skin: The application area should be clean, dry, and free of any oils, lotions, or perspiration. Even natural skin oils can interfere with adhesion, so a quick wipe with a damp cloth or alcohol swab is recommended.

- Avoid Hairy Areas: If possible, choose areas with minimal hair for better adhesion. For individuals with delicate skin, placing the patch on a less sensitive and less hairy region can help alleviate any discomfort during removal.
- Adjust Positioning: Modifying the positioning slightly each day aids in avoiding skin discomfort. For patches that require daily application, like the Energy Enhancer, alternating between the left and right sides of the body or varying the acupressure points can be advantageous.

2. Comprehensive Guidelines for Each Patch

Every LifeWave patch comes with tailored instructions for ideal placement, crafted to correspond with its unique function. Here's a comprehensive analysis for each category:

IceWave Patch: Alleviating Discomfort and Reducing Swelling

- Primary Placement Points: IceWave patches are usually positioned on the painful area using a dual patch technique. The patches are available in a pair (one white and one tan), typically with the white patch positioned on the right side and the tan patch on the left.

- Alternative Points: If direct placement isn't effective, the patches can be applied to different locations, such as on the wrists or the back of the knees. These regions align with specific points for alleviating discomfort.
- Layering: Users can apply an Aeon patch alongside IceWave for enhanced relief from stress or inflammation. In this scenario, Aeon can be positioned on a wrist point, while IceWave patches can be strategically placed close to the area experiencing discomfort.

Energy Enhancer Patch: Elevating Vitality and Endurance

- Primary Placement Points: The Energy Enhancer patch is typically positioned on specific points of the body, such as the chest or lower extremities, including the wrists or just above the ankles, with the white patch placed on the right side and the tan patch on the left side.
- Optional Points for Vitality: Some individuals choose to apply these on areas close to muscle groups or regions that feel tired, like the shoulders or lower back, to enhance endurance in those specific areas.
- Layering: To boost vitality and concentration, the Energy Enhancer can be paired with a Silent Nights patch applied to the back of the neck for a soothing effect.

Aeon Patch: Alleviating Tension and Promoting Calmness

- Primary Placement Points: Aeon patches are effective when applied to areas that impact stress responses, including the wrist, neck, or behind the ear. These areas can assist in harmonizing the nervous system.
- Additional Placement Options: Some users apply the Aeon patch on the forehead or crown of the head, as these areas are linked to enhanced mental clarity and tranquility in traditional practices.
- Layering: Aeon complements patches such as Silent Nights for individuals seeking a synergistic effect on relaxation and sleep enhancement. In this pairing, Aeon can be applied to the wrist or the back of the neck, while Silent Nights is positioned on another suggested area for sleep enhancement.

Silent Nights Patch: Restful Sleep Aid

- Primary Placement Points: Silent Nights is typically positioned on the temple or just behind the ear to facilitate the onset of sleep. These regions are adjacent to points that encourage restful sleep through acupressure techniques.
- Alternative Placement: Individuals who find this position uncomfortable can also position Silent Nights on the bottom of

the foot, near the ball, which serves as an effective pressure point for promoting restful sleep.
- Layering: To improve sleep quality, individuals might use Aeon for stress reduction during the day and transition to Silent Nights as bedtime approaches.

Y-Age Carnosine Patch: Promoting Skin and Wound Recovery

- Optimal Placement Areas: Carnosine patches are most effective when positioned close to the targeted area, like directly over a scar or adjacent to a wound to promote skin recovery. Typical placements include the chest area or just below the navel, as these sites are believed to stimulate restorative functions.
- Alternative Points for Healing: Pressure points located on the back, especially along the spine, provide valuable support for overall tissue health.
- Layering: When combining with other Y-Age patches like Glutathione, it's optimal to place them in supportive locations, such as one on the wrist and the other on the chest.

Glutathione Patch: Enhancing Detoxification and Strengthening Immunity

- Primary Placement Points: These patches are typically placed on the upper chest or just below the navel. These areas are perfect for cleansing, as they align with energy points related to immunity in traditional Chinese practices.
- Additional Points: Users may also apply these on areas linked to fluid movement, such as the lower back or inner elbow.
- Layering: Combining glutathione with the Energy Enhancer or Aeon patch can enhance overall wellness. When applying layers, position Glutathione near the torso and place Energy Enhancer closer to the extremities.

Nirvana Patch: Elevating Your Mood

- Primary Placement Points: The Nirvana patch is usually positioned close to the heart or on the wrist, focusing on areas associated with emotional equilibrium and mood management.
- Additional Points: Users can place the Nirvana patch behind the ear or on the temple to enhance their mood further.
- Layering: For holistic mood enhancement, Nirvana can be applied in conjunction with Aeon at a separate location to target stress and emotional equilibrium.

SP6 Complete Patch: Appetite Regulation

- Primary Placement Points: SP6 Complete is typically positioned on the ankle, particularly at the point associated with appetite management and metabolic balance.
- Additional Placement Options: Users can explore points around the abdomen or wrists, as these regions relate to appetite regulation and hormonal equilibrium.
- Layering: Using SP6 Complete alongside the Energy Enhancer or Aeon patch can promote metabolic wellness and alleviate stress while also aiding in appetite management.

Using LifeWave patches correctly and regularly can lead to the best health outcomes. Every patch is designed with distinct placement points and detailed instructions to engage the body's inherent healing and energy mechanisms. Adhering to these comprehensive application instructions will enable users to maximize the benefits of their patches, whether their goal is alleviating discomfort, boosting energy, promoting relaxation, or enhancing sleep quality.

CHAPTER 5

Guidelines for Optimal Application of LifeWave Patches

To fully harness the advantages of LifeWave patches, it's essential to follow several key steps: define your health objectives, comprehend the optimal placement of the patches, rotate them as necessary, and monitor your progress effectively. This guide provides practical training strategies to maximize the benefits of LifeWave's innovative, phototherapy-based patches.

1. Grasping Indicators and Objectives

When beginning with LifeWave patches, it's essential to have a precise grasp of your wellness goals. Each patch is crafted to address particular requirements, allowing you to choose them more efficiently by concentrating on symptoms and intended results.

Defining Wellness Objectives

Wellness objectives can encompass a variety of aspects, including physical improvements like alleviating discomfort or boosting vitality, as well as emotional and mental health enhancements such as better sleep patterns or effective stress management. Here's a detailed guide on how to tackle each aspect:

- Pain Relief: If alleviating discomfort is your objective, you might want to explore the IceWave patch, recognized for its effectiveness in providing relief. Furthermore, if inflammation or stress

intensifies the discomfort, the Aeon patch may serve as a beneficial addition.
- Vitality and Endurance: To boost vitality and enhance physical endurance, the Vitality Booster patch is perfect. Numerous individuals discover it especially beneficial when energy requirements vary during the day or to enhance stamina during physical exertion.
- Stress and Relaxation: If you're looking to alleviate stress, the Aeon patch is crafted to promote relaxation and enhance mental clarity. Numerous individuals discover it beneficial to utilize alongside other patches such as Silent Nights to enhance restorative sleep.
- Sleep Support: Individuals experiencing difficulties with sleep may want to explore the Silent Nights patch, which aids in enhancing sleep quality in a natural way. Combining it with the Aeon patch throughout the day can help manage stress that could disrupt relaxation.
- Detoxification and Immunity: The Glutathione patch is advantageous for individuals seeking to cleanse their system or enhance their immune response. This patch operates efficiently in consistent intervals and can enhance overall well-being, particularly during transitions in seasons or following an illness.
- Skin and Tissue Repair: The Y-Age Carnosine patch supports the healing of

skin and tissue, making it beneficial for individuals recovering from minor injuries or looking to enhance their skin health.

Aligning Patches with Manifestations

Each individual's body reacts uniquely, and monitoring your particular symptoms will assist in choosing the right patches. For instance, if you observe that tiredness is accompanied by stress, combining Energy Enhancer with Aeon might yield more harmonious outcomes. Over time, as you learn which symptoms respond best to certain patches, you'll be able to customize your approach more effectively.

2. Techniques for Patch Placement

Proper placement of LifeWave patches can significantly impact their effectiveness. While each patch has recommended points, learning alternative placements can enhance your results.

Primary and Secondary Placement Points

- Primary Points: These are the recommended placements that correspond with acupressure or meridian points. Each patch's primary points are designed to achieve the most consistent

results, based on research and user feedback.
- Secondary or Alternative Points: Many users find secondary points helpful when primary placements aren't convenient or when they're layering multiple patches. Alternative placements are often located on the wrists, ankles, or spine. For example:
- Energy Enhancer: Typically applied above the ankles, this patch can also be placed on the wrists or shoulders for additional stimulation of energy points.
- Silent Nights: Generally placed on the temple or behind the ear, Silent Nights can be applied on the back of the neck for more subtle support in improving sleep quality.

Exploring Placement Methods

To get the best experience with LifeWave patches, consider these placement methods:

- Balance for Pain Relief: With IceWave patches, achieving balance can make a difference. Position the white patch on one side of the discomfort zone and the tan patch on the opposite side. This technique establishes equilibrium in light therapy around the area of discomfort.
- Rotational Placement: Changing patch placement every few days prevents skin irritation and can help prevent your body

from adapting to a single location. For instance, Energy Enhancer can be worn on the right wrist one day and the left ankle the next.
- Tracking Responses: Keep track of which placements feel the most effective. Some people respond better to less common points, such as the inner elbow or spine. Recording this helps personalize your patch routine.

3. Integration and Movement

LifeWave patches offer flexibility in their application, enabling you to combine or alternate them based on your specific requirements, thereby facilitating the management of various symptoms or objectives as needed. Understanding how to skillfully integrate and alternate patches is essential for achieving equilibrium and enhancing advantages.

Integrating Patches for Enhanced Advantages

Employing various patches can effectively tackle intricate challenges, including tension and exhaustion. However, merging patches should be approached with care to prevent excessive stimulation of your body.

- Synergistic Patches: Certain patches collaborate effectively to produce holistic outcomes. For example:
- Energy and Stress Management: Combine the Energy Enhancer patch with Aeon for optimal results. This blend is beneficial for individuals seeking an energy lift while navigating stress levels.
- Pain and Relaxation: Utilizing IceWave alongside Aeon effectively addresses the pain directly while also alleviating the stress that may intensify it.
- Rest and Purification: Combining restful nights with Glutathione can enhance sleep quality and promote daily cleansing, aiding in overall recovery and rejuvenation.

Utilizing Rotating Patches for Reliable Outcomes

Incorporating rotation is advantageous when applying patches consistently over a prolonged duration. Switching between various areas enables you to target diverse objectives and provides your body with an opportunity to adapt.

- Weekly Rotation: For instance, you could utilize Energy Enhancer throughout the week, transition to Glutathione on the weekends, and add Aeon for stress management on especially tough days.
- Short Breaks: Taking a one- or two-day break each week aids in recalibrating the

body's reactions. A significant number of individuals report experiencing enhanced effects following a short break in usage.
- Monitoring the Advantages of Rotation: Observe how your body reacts to various patches during rotation. This aids in pinpointing the patches that are most advantageous for particular symptoms or requirements, and can guide future application trends.

4. Monitoring Outcomes

To maximize the benefits of LifeWave patches, monitoring is essential. Documenting your experiences with each patch and its placement will assist you in discovering what is most effective for your body.
Developing a Record of Indicators, Uses, and Outcomes

A straightforward journal serves as an excellent tool for monitoring your LifeWave patch application. Every entry may encompass information regarding symptoms, the positioning of patches, and the results that have been noted.

- Daily Symptoms: Record any sensations you're encountering, including tiredness, tension, discomfort, or difficulties with sleep. This assists you in choosing the most suitable patch for each day.

- Application of the Patch: Document the locations of each patch application, the duration of wear, and any differences in placement. This approach allows you to observe which regions of the body exhibit the most significant responses.
- Instant and Lasting Outcomes: Some effects, such as relief from discomfort, can be experienced rapidly, while others, like enhanced vitality or improved rest, might require a bit more time to manifest. Document both immediate responses and ongoing trends over several weeks to observe how regular engagement influences your overall well-being.

Recognizing Trends and Modifying Application

By monitoring patch usage and symptoms, you will begin to observe trends that can guide your future applications. For example:

- Identifying Key Areas of Impact: You might discover that specific areas yield the most significant results. These patches can be emphasized for regular application.
- Seasonal or Situational Adjustments: Over time, you may discover that particular patches provide greater benefits during certain times of the year or in specific circumstances (e.g.,

Glutathione in colder months, Silent Nights during times of stress).
- Enhancing Patch Positioning: Analyzing your notes can uncover the most effective areas for specific patches, enabling you to refine your strategy.

Monitoring Comprehensive Health

LifeWave patches aim to enhance comprehensive well-being, making it important to monitor your overall health as well. Observe any shifts in mood, energy levels, or digestive health, as light therapy can influence various aspects of the body's functioning. This comprehensive tracking method enables you to observe the complete effects that LifeWave patches have on your overall health and wellness.

Mastering the effective application of LifeWave patches demands a careful strategy, informed by your symptoms, aspirations, and individual experiences. By following these suggestions, you can choose the most suitable patches, enhance their positioning, blend them for optimal advantage, and maintain a log of your outcomes. This comprehensive method will enable you to thoroughly engage and modify your practices to optimally enhance your wellness journey with LifeWave.

CHAPTER 6

Guidelines and Optimal Approaches for LifeWave Patch Application

LifeWave patches aim to enhance health and well-being, yet proper application is crucial to optimize their advantages and reduce the potential for irritation or negative reactions. This guide outlines essential safety measures, usage protocols, and optimal techniques to guarantee a successful and pleasant experience. Adhering to these methods can improve outcomes while ensuring you remain mindful and attuned to your body's reactions to the patches.

1. Essential Safety Protocols

When utilizing LifeWave patches, it is crucial to comprehend the appropriate duration for wearing them and to avoid excessive use. Adhering to these recommendations can help avoid skin sensitivity and enhance your overall experience.

Length of Time for Each Session of Patch Application

Every LifeWave patch is crafted to be utilized for a designated duration to enhance its advantages while ensuring the body is not overstressed. Below are the standard recommendations for the duration of patch use:

- Daily Limit: LifeWave suggests using the patches for a maximum of 12 hours in any given 24-hour timeframe. Prolonged use may elevate the likelihood of skin irritation, especially in delicate regions.
- Night-Time Usage: For patches designed to enhance sleep, such as Silent Nights, it is best to wear them throughout the night and take them off upon waking. This offers the advantages for sleep without prolonged use that could lead to skin problems.
- Alternate Days: Should you notice increased sensitivity, consider applying the patches on alternate days. This approach can help avoid excessive stimulation and allow your body the necessary time to adapt to the effects.
- Rest Intervals: Allowing yourself one or two days of rest each week from patch usage can be advantageous, particularly for individuals who have been using them consistently for several weeks. This period of rest enables the body to rejuvenate, frequently resulting in a more pronounced impact when activities are resumed.

Preventing Excessive Use and Reliance

Excessive use of any wellness tool, such as LifeWave patches, may diminish its efficacy and result in tolerance. To prevent this:

- Adhere to Suggested Protocols: Maintaining the advised duration and frequency helps prevent excessive strain on your body. Excessive use does not improve advantages and can lead to adaptation, reducing outcomes.
- Refrain from Stacking Multiple Patches of the Same Type: Applying more than one of the same patch type, like two Energy Enhancers, is typically unnecessary and could even be counterproductive. Instead, position one patch in an area that can yield the best advantages.

Skin Care Precautions

Since LifeWave patches are applied directly to the skin, caring for the application site is important to prevent any discomfort or irritation:

- Clean and Dry the Skin: Always apply patches to clean, dry skin. Oils, lotions, or sweat can prevent proper adhesion and interfere with patch effectiveness.
- Rotate Application Sites: Rotating where you place patches on your body

can help reduce irritation from prolonged use in the same area. Try switching the patch from your right wrist to your left wrist or another location the following day.
- Observe Skin Responses: Should you notice any redness or sensitivity where the patch was applied, take it off and allow the area to recover. Minor reactions typically subside swiftly, yet ongoing discomfort could suggest a sensitivity to the adhesive.

2. Addressing Skin Sensitivities and Alleviating Irritation

LifeWave patches are crafted to be gentle on the skin; nonetheless, a few individuals might still encounter sensitivity. Here's a guide to recognizing and addressing possible skin responses.

Indicators of Skin Sensitivity

Skin sensitivity can manifest in several typical forms:

- Redness or Itching: This may occur if the skin reacts to the adhesive or if the patch is used beyond the suggested duration.
- Dryness or Peeling: Prolonged application on a single area may lead to dryness; varying the application sites can help mitigate this issue.

- Elevated, Inflamed Skin: If the skin appears elevated or shows signs of inflammation, it could suggest an allergic response. In such instances, it is essential to take off the patch right away.

Addressing and Averting Discomfort

If you encounter slight skin sensitivity, following these steps may alleviate irritation:

- Utilize Diverse Regions: Switching between multiple suggested regions can assist in avoiding excessive sensitivity in any one area. For instance, if one wrist experiences discomfort, consider trying the opposite wrist or ankle.
- Utilize a Protective Layer: Placing a slender protective layer, such as medical-grade tape or hypoallergenic adhesive, between the patch and the skin may benefit those with sensitivities. Ensure that the barrier does not disrupt the patch's effectiveness.
- Reduce Wear Time: If discomfort arises despite correct positioning, shortening the duration of use might be beneficial. Begin by using the patch for six to eight hours rather than the full 12, and slowly increase the duration if it feels comfortable.
- Use a Gentle Moisturizer: Following the removal of the patch, applying a gentle,

fragrance-free lotion can help calm the skin.

When to Consult a Healthcare Professional

While most skin reactions are minor, any persistent discomfort should be discussed with a healthcare provider, especially for individuals with pre-existing skin conditions like eczema or psoriasis.

3. Who Should Avoid Using LifeWave Patches

LifeWave patches are generally safe for most people. However, certain individuals should exercise caution or consult with a healthcare provider before using them.

Considerations for Particular Health Issues

Some health conditions might necessitate careful consideration when utilizing LifeWave patches:

- Pregnancy and Breastfeeding: Given the limited research on the impact of phototherapy patches during pregnancy or lactation, it is advisable for those who are pregnant or breastfeeding to refrain

from using LifeWave patches unless directed by a healthcare provider.
- Pacemakers or Implanted Medical Devices: Those with pacemakers or similar implanted devices are advised to seek guidance from a healthcare professional, as there may be potential electromagnetic interference from external devices.
- Chronic Skin Conditions: Individuals with skin sensitivities or ongoing conditions (like eczema, psoriasis, or dermatitis) should approach the use of patches with caution, as these conditions may heighten the risk of skin irritation.
- Individuals with Allergies: While LifeWave patches are designed to be hypoallergenic, those who are sensitive to adhesives or prone to allergic reactions might still encounter some discomfort. It is recommended to observe the skin attentively.

Factors Related to Age

- Youth and Teens: LifeWave patches are mainly intended for grown-ups. When applied to younger individuals, it is essential that a healthcare professional oversees the process, and the duration of application should typically be reduced to accommodate their smaller physiques.
- Elderly Individuals: Elderly individuals with delicate or thinning skin should exercise caution regarding the placement

and duration. It is advisable to use patches for limited durations while monitoring skin responses.

4. Storage and Maintenance of Patches

Correctly storing LifeWave patches guarantees their efficacy is maintained over time. Given that patches depend on particular materials and technology, inadequate storage may result in reduced effectiveness.

Guidelines for Patch Storage

- Maintain Sealed Packaging: LifeWave patches are provided in sealed packaging to ensure their optimal effectiveness. Maintain their sealed state until needed to avoid contact with air and humidity.
- Keep in a Cool, Dry Environment: Ensure patches are not subjected to excessive heat, direct sunlight, or moisture. Keep them in a drawer or cabinet at room temperature, ensuring they are away from windows, heat sources, and damp areas.
- Minimize Contact: Frequent touching of the adhesive side of the patch can diminish its adherence and potentially compromise its overall performance. When applying patches, make sure to only touch the edges.
Verifying Expiration Dates

LifeWave patches have expiration dates, and utilizing them beyond this point could diminish their efficacy. Outdated patches might diminish in their stickiness or effectiveness, so it's essential to verify the dates prior to usage.

Advice for Traveling and Using While Mobile

For those who want to carry LifeWave patches while on the move, here are some tips to ensure their protection:

- Travel Containers: It's a good idea to store some patches in a compact, airtight container, particularly when journeying through humid or warm environments. This aids in shielding them from moisture or extreme temperatures.
- Pre-Cut and Ready: For those with a busy lifestyle, preparing a patch pack in advance can be advantageous, providing swift access when it's time to apply.
- Maintain a Comfortable Temperature: When visiting hot locations, consider keeping patches in a cooler bag when they are not being used.

Ensuring safety is essential for maximizing the benefits of LifeWave patches. By adhering to these recommendations—like minimizing duration of use, alternating application areas, monitoring skin reactions, and applying as instructed—you can seamlessly incorporate LifeWave patches into your health and wellness regimen. Properly storing patches and being aware of any health precautions or contraindications are crucial steps in achieving safe, effective, and optimal results with LifeWave products. Implementing these optimal strategies, while being mindful of personal reactions, can enhance your results and lead to a more reliable and rewarding experience with LifeWave patches.

THE END